I0435048

Paleo Chicken Crockpot Cookbook

Easy and Delicious American, Italian, Mexican, and Asian Recipes

Contents

About the Book

This book is for people wanting to follow the Paleo diet, which is based on the diets of our caveman ancestors. The diet includes all-natural foods which can be either hunted or gathered. This book contains recipes that feature chicken as the main ingredient.

Find slow cooked crockpot recipes that marinate the chicken in a variety of flavors. It is organized into four sections based on various cuisines from around the world i.e. Asian, Mexican, Italian and American styles. The nutritional approach doesn't compromise delicious taste and offers incredible flavors, variety and health benefits. Enjoy a variation of flavors from different cultures all in one easy to prepare and easy to clean crockpot.

Introduction

This book includes delicious and nutritious Paleo recipes featuring Chicken. The Paleo diet, also known as the caveman diet or Stone Age diet, is a nutritional plan based on food groups preferred by our ancestors during the Paleolithic era. The foods included in this group are fresh meats (beef, poultry, lamb, and pork), seafood, fish, fresh fruits, nuts, vegetables, seeds and healthy oils (like olive, coconut, etc.)

The recipes contain loads of lean proteins, fiber, healthy fats, minerals and vitamins. By including Paleo in daily eating, many health benefits may be achieved. The Paleo diet helps in weight loss and muscle growth while keeping an active lifestyle. Other benefits of the Paleo diet include improved metabolism, better sleep, a healthy ratio of Omega 3: Omega 6 fatty acids, stable blood sugar levels, reduced allergies, clearer skin and improved mood. The diet also lowers the risk of heart disease, diabetes, cancer, immune system deficiencies and asthma. Enjoy the aromas and delicious flavors of these dishes after they slowly cook in the crockpot for hours.

Asian Style

Chicken wings

Servings: 4-6

1 Kg Chicken wings

1/2 cup melted grass-fed ghee

1/2 cup red hot sauce

1/2 tsp paprika

1/2 tsp salt

1/4 cup apple cider vinegar

1/4 tsp black pepper

Preheat the oven on broil about 10 min. Place your chicken in the broiler for about 5 min. per side, to make it crispy. Melt your grass-fed ghee and then add red hot sauce, paprika, apple cider vinegar, black pepper and salt to it. Grease your Crockpot. Place your crispy chicken in the crockpot. Spread all sauce on the wings and mix to make the wings saucy. Cook for 2 hours. Carefully stir up the sauce and wings once or twice during cooking time. Serve hot and enjoy Paleo Hot wings in simple way.

Indian Chicken Curry

Servings: 6-8

1 kg boneless chicken breast, diced

200 ml chicken broth

500 ml of coconut milk

3 tsp red curry paste

1 small yellow onion

1/2 medium red bell pepper

3 cloves garlic

¼ head of cabbage

¼ head of cauliflower

Before starting the preparation, set the crockpot on low. Pour chicken broth and coconut milk into the crockpot and add curry paste. Dissolve it properly. Cut the chicken, onion and red pepper into 1"cubes. Place them all into crockpot and stir. Chop up the cauliflower into florets and the cabbage into thin strips. Add both into pot and stir. Mince garlic and add it in. After adding all ingredients, cover the pot and let it cook for 4 hrs on low. Then serve!

Indian Grass-fed ghee Chicken

Servings 4-6

1 Kg Boneless Chicken

1 diced onion

6 minced garlic cloves

4-6 tsp grass-fed ghee

15 cardamom pods (sewn together in a tea bag)

2 tsp garam masala

2 tsp curry powder

1/8 tsp cayenne pepper

1 pinch ground ginger

200 ml coconut milk

100 ml tomato paste

2 tsp lemon juice

Put the chicken in your crockpot. Pack your cardamom in a tea bag and place it aside. (Because we want only the flavor of cardamom, not exact cardamom. we add it in a tea bag and after cooking we easily remove and discard it.) Add all the ingredients to the crockpot and mix well together with a rubber spatula. Carefully add the cardamom bag at the end and submerge it in liquid. Cook for 8 hrs. on low or for 4-5 hrs. on high heat. Discard the cardamom bag. Shred the chicken a little bit and soak in the liquid. Serve in bowl.

Chinese Honey Sesame Chicken

Servings: 3

6-8 chicken thighs (approx. 1 Kg)

salt to taste

1 small onion (diced)

1/4 cup tomato paste

3 cloves garlic (minced)

1 tsp freshly ground black pepper

1/2 cup gluten free soy sauce

1 cup honey

1/2 tsp red chili paste

2 tsp sesame seeds

Plop your chicken thighs in the crockpot. Sprinkle some black pepper and salt on top. Leaving out the sesame seeds, mix all the ingredients together in a bowl. Pour this mixture on the chicken thighs. Cook on low heat for 7-8 hrs and then remove the cover and cook further for about 15 min to thicken the liquid. This dish has a lot of liquid. If you want it less watery then evaporate to your liking. Spread sesame seeds before serving. Serve with steamed cauliflower and broccoli.

Japanese Ginger Lime Chicken

Servings: 3

500gm boneless chicken

1 inch ginger (grated)

2 cloves garlic

Pinch of turmeric

4 tsp cilantro

½ green bell pepper

6 tsp olive oil

4 tsp garam masala

2 green chillies

1 small onion

Lime wedges

Salt

Chop cilantro. Grate chicken. Put ginger, garlic, onion, turmeric, cilantro, bell pepper, garam masala, green chilies and salt into a food processor and chop it. Mix the chicken into it and mix it well. Remove and shape into 16-20 balls. Grease your crockpot and spread the rounds into it. Cook on low for about 4 hrs. Serve hot with lime wedges or Paleo friendly salsa.

Thai Coconut Chicken Soup

Servings: 4-5

½ Kg boneless, skinless chicken thighs

4 cups chicken broth

400 ml coconut milk

3 medium sized tomatoes

5-6 small sweet bell peppers

250 gm mushrooms

5 tsp lime juice

3 tsp fish sauce

1 tsp chili paste

3-4 cloves garlic, diced

1 inch ginger freshly grated

Seafood (optional)

Mix chicken broth, coconut milk, lime juice, fish sauce, chili paste, ginger and garlic together in the crockpot. This is your soup base. Chop your vegetables in bigger chunks or as you prefer. Cut up the chicken and add it to the base. Add your veggies too. Cook on low heat for 4-5 hrs. If you are using seafood, then add it in during the last 30 min. You can make variations as per your choice. Fried seafood has its own delicious taste with chicken soup.

Almond Chicken Thighs

Servings: 2-3

4 boneless, skinless chicken thighs (or chicken breasts)

1/2 cups chicken broth

1 tsp olive oil

8-12 large olives

1/2 cup whole raw almonds

1 cloves garlic

1/4 onion, coarsely chopped

1/2 tsp chili powder

1/4 tsp black pepper

1/2 tsp cumin

Grease your crockpot with the olive oil. Mix all ingredients in a mixing bowl and then add in the chicken. Place all content in crockpot. Cook for 8 hrs on low heat. Serve with roasted grass-fed gheenut squash.

Mexican Style

Spicy Cilantro Crockpot chicken

Servings: 4-6

1 whole chicken (about 2 Kg)

1 tsp Black pepper

2 tsp chilli powder

1 tsp cayenne powder

1 ½ tsp ground cumin

1 tsp Sea salt

½ cup lime juice

1 lime (whole)

1 cup fresh cilantro, chopped

1 tsp olive oil

4 cloves garlic

Wash and dry the whole chicken. Rub salt and pepper on it. Mix chili powder, cayenne, and cumin. Cover the chicken completely. Now make a fine paste of chili powder, cayenne, and cumin in a blender. Keep the whole lime in the cavity of your chicken. Poke lots of holes into chicken using a fork. Transfer it into a marinating bag.. Add in the paste. Make sure that the marinade is applied under the skin also. Let your chicken marinate overnight. Add the chicken to the crockpot in the morning and cook on low for 6-8 hrs. Check if it is done, remove from the pot and enjoy.

Mexican Chicken Stuffed Peppers

Servings: 2

4 large bell peppers

3 chicken breast

1 cup diced tomatoes

½ cup tomato juice

2 tsp chopped jalapenos

¼ cup chopped green peppers

¼ cup minced onion

2 cup Paleo salsa

1 tsp ground cumin

¼ tsp oregano

½ tsp garlic powder

½ tsp crushed red pepper

1 tsp chili powder

1 tsp salt

2 tsp onion powder

Put your chicken breasts and all spices into the crockpot. Mix it well and cook on low for 6-7 hrs. When the chicken is done. Remove it from the pot and shred it using two forks. Mix it back in. Take your bell pepper and cut the top of pepper off and pull out the ribs and seeds. Wash it and stuff peppers with shredded chicken. Put some Paleo salsa on top and bake for 20 min at 350. The peppers will soften. Garnish with some more salsa and its ready to eat.

Shredded Mexican Crock-Pot Chicken

Servings: 2-3

4 chicken breasts

1 tsp. cumin

1 tbsp. powdered chili

1/2 tsp. ground coriander

1/4 tsp. smoked paprika

1 1/2 tsp. sea salt

1/2 tsp. ground pepper

1/3 c. broth

1/3 c. cilantro, chopped

1 lime

1 yellow onion, chop

1 jalapeno, Remove seeds and mince

4 cloves of garlic, mince

1 tbsp. olive oil

Heat up the olive oil in a medium sauté pan. Stir in the onions and sauté until translucent. Sprinkle in the cumin, powder, coriander, paprika and cloves combine and stir for about 3 minutes. Pour the chicken broth into the pan. Season the chicken breasts with salt to taste and pepper. Then transfer to the crock pot. Squeeze lime juice in and mix in the remaining ingredients. Cook on low for 3-5 hours. Remove chicken from the crock pot, shred and place in a bowl. Add this chicken to a bowl and garnish with shredded cilantro and jalapeno.

Crock Pot Mexican Chicken Soup

Servings: 6

1 whole chicken, divided into parts

6 cups chicken broth

½ yellow onion, chopped

1 pepper, chopped

3 carrots, sliced

3 tomatoes, chopped

4 garlic cloves, sliced

1 tsp cumin

1 cup tomato juice

1 tsp ground coriander

½ cup cilantro

2 tsp sea salt

Juice of 2 limes

Put chicken, chicken broth, onion, pepper, carrots, tomatoes, garlic, cumin, tomato juice, coriander and salt into a crockpot. Cover and cook for 6 hrs. on low or 3 hrs. on high. Remove only the chicken and shred it. Discard the bones and put the chicken back in the pot. Add lime juice and chopped cilantro. Continue cooking for 1 hr more. Your Mexican style crockpot chicken soup is ready to serve.

Fresh Crockpot Mexican Chicken Tacos

Servings: 4-6

1 kg boneless skinless chicken breast

1 cup chicken broth

1/3 c. Paleo salsa

1 can diced green chills

1/2 tsp onion powder

1/2 tsp garlic powder

1/8 tsp chili powder

1/4 tsp paprika

1 1/2 tsp cumin

sea salt and pepper to taste

Grass-fed ghee Lettuce

fresh cilantro - chopped

lime juice

Place chicken in the crockpot. Add all remaining ingredients first mixing them together in separate bowl. When well combined, transfer to the crockpot. Cook on high for 6-8 hours. Shred the chicken 30 min before serving and allow juices to soak into the meat. Wash grass-fed ghee lettuce and prepare toppings. Make little tacos using the lettuce as your wrap. Top with little fresh cilantro. Put all "tacos" on a plate and squeeze some lime on top!

Italian Style

Oregano Spinach Chicken

Servings: 4-6

1 Kg chicken thigh

8 cloves garlic

½ cup balsamic vinegar

250 gm.. baby Spinach

2 tsp. oregano

½ tsp. black pepper

2 tsp. parsley

Place your chicken thighs in crockpot. Mix all ingredients except the spinach and pour it on the chicken thighs. Cook your chicken for 6-7 hrs. on low heat and 3-4 hrs. on high heat. Add spinach on the top and cook further for 15 min. Serve hot.

Simple Crockpot Italian Chicken

Servings: 4-6

6-8 boneless chicken breasts

1 c. diced tomatoes, drained

1 1/2 cups chicken broth

1 tsp. Italian herbs seasoning

2 tsp. extra virgin olive oil

2 garlic cloves, mashed

Sea salt and pepper to taste

Grease your crockpot with virgin olive oil and spread your chicken breasts in the bottom of pot. Add garlic cloves, Italian seasoning, pepper and sea salt into it. Pour chicken broth and diced tomatoes in chicken. Mix it together well. Cook for 4-5 hrs. on low heat and your crockpot Italian chicken is ready to serve.

Creamy Italian Chicken Tomato Soup

Servings: 6-8

3 large boneless skinless chicken breasts

1 cup chicken broth

1 small onion, chopped

2 cloves garlic, minced

1 can coconut milk (full fat)

1 can diced tomatoes

1 can tomato sauce

2 tsp. Italian herbs seasoning

1 tsp. dried basil

1/2 tsp sea salt

Fresh ground pepper to taste

Mix coconut milk, chicken broth, tomato sauce, and diced tomatoes along with the seasonings in your crock pot. Add chicken. Cover and cook on low for 7-9 hours or on high for 4-6 hours .Shred chicken and return to crock pot. Keep warm until ready to serve.

Lemon Garlic Crockpot Chicken

Servings: 4

1 whole chicken

2 tsp. Italian herbs seasoning

7 cloves of garlic, peeled

1 whole lemon

1 white onion, sliced

Salt and pepper

Take a clean whole chicken. Season it with pepper, salt and Italian blend on both the inside and outside. Squeeze juice of a half lemon on the chicken, place half the lemon inside the chicken's cavity and set it aside. Spread sliced onion and peeled garlic cloves at the bottom of your crockpot. Put your seasoned chicken on them, cover and cook for 6 hrs. over low heat. Remove the cooked chicken and shred it with forks. Then place back the shredded chicken, mix well with onion and garlic and enjoy!

Crock Pot Italian Herb Meat Balls

Servings: 4

600gm ground chicken

¼ cup chopped of Italian Parsley

2 eggs

2 tsp dried minced onion flakes

1 tsp garlic powder

½ tsp sea salt

½ tsp ground black pepper

1 cup Almond flour

2 cups chicken broth

1 can tomato paste

In a big mixing bowl, combine the chopped parsley with the ground chicken. Add in the eggs, and the dried spices and mix them well using your hands. After the chicken is mixed thoroughly, roll it into golf ball sized balls. Once you have the chicken balls all rolled up, go ahead and roll the chicken balls into the almond flour. Place them in your crock pot. Mix the 2 cups of broth with the tomato paste and pour over the meatballs and cook for 8-10 hours on low.

Italian Crock Pot Chili

Servings: 6-8

½ kg ground chicken

1 onion, chopped

100gm baby Bella mushrooms, diced

1 can fire-roasted diced tomatoes

1 tsp minced garlic

3-4 tsp capers

1/4 small can of tomato paste

1-2 c chicken broth

3 bay leaves

2 tsp dried thyme

2 tsp dried basil

2 tsp chili powder

1 tsp cayenne

2-3 tsp balsamic vinegar

Salt and pepper to taste

Drizzle of olive oil

Place all the ground chicken in the crock pot along with salt, pepper and one chopped onion, until they become brown. Turn the crock pot on low and cook for 3-4 hours, stirring occasionally. After your chicken is done and drained, add the mushrooms, tomatoes, capers, garlic, and tomato paste. Stir and then add the remaining ingredients and mix thoroughly. Cook on low for 3 hrs or until the veggies are done. Serve with diced avocado on top.

Italian Herb Chicken Stew

Servings: 6

12 Boneless, skinless chicken thighs

1 Onion, chopped finely

1 can Fire roasted, diced Tomatoes

1 cup Mushrooms

1/2 can Tomato paste

2-3 Carrots, chopped

3 stalks Celery, chopped

1-2 tsp Coconut oil

4 cloves Garlic, minced

1 tsp dry Basil

1 tsp. Italian herb seasoning

1 cup full fat coconut cream

Salt &Pepper to taste

Take a frying pan, heat the coconut oil first. Then add in the onions, carrots and celery and fry for 5 min. In a bowl add mushrooms, tomato paste, basil, garlic and the herb seasoning blend, mix it well. Cut the chicken into small cubes. Take a crockpot and spread the carrot mixture in the bottom, then add mushroom mixture from the bowl, then add the chicken cubes. Pour tomatoes and coconut milk over it. Stir and cook on high for 4 hrs. Add pepper and salt. Splash a little coconut cream on top before serving.

American Style

Roasted, Orange Infused Chicken

Servings: 4

1 whole chicken

2 tsp olive oil

1/2 orange

1 whole onion

4 garlic cloves

3 whole celery ribs

4 whole carrots

1 tsp fresh thyme

1 tsp kosher salt

1 tsp black pepper

Cut the onion, celery and carrots up and put them in the bottom of your crock pot. You are not going to eat these with the chicken; they stay there for making stock. Putting them in the bottom of the crock pot keeps the chicken elevated out of the juice and lets the chicken roast instead of stew. Combine the garlic cloves, olive oil, salt, and pepper. Add about 1/2 tsp of the fresh thyme leaves. Take the garlic paste and spread it under the skin of the chicken. Try not to poke holes in the skin. Make sure you flavor the breasts and thighs. Stuff the orange and fresh thyme in the cavity of the chicken. Roast in your crock pot for 3 to 4 hours on High. Remove chicken, serve and enjoy.

Crockpot Portobello Chickens

Servings: 2

2 small chickens

2 large portabella mushrooms

2 medium onions

1 garlic bulb

1 lemon

2 tsp combined herbs and spices of choice

2 tsp olive oil

Rinse, pat dry, and season the baby/ small chickens. Grease the crockpot. Place the mushrooms in the crockpot; keep the stem side up in the crockpot. Slice and layer the onions over the mushrooms. Sprinkle roughly chopped garlic over the onions. Cut the lemon in half and stuff each chicken with both a garlic and a lemon half inside the cavity and place them breast side down inside the crockpot. Cook halfway for 2 ½ hrs on high, remove cover and turn chickens over and finish cooking later for 2 ½ hrs.

Honey Rotisserie Chicken

Servings: 4

1 whole chicken

1 tsp honey

1/4 cup paprika

1/2 tsp salt

1 tsp celery salt

1 tsp ground black pepper

1/2 tsp cayenne pepper

1 tsp dry mustard

1 tsp garlic powder

1 tsp onion powder

Aluminum foil

Roll aluminum foil into balls (8-9, about 1 inch each) and add to bottom of your crockpot. Rinse and pat dry the whole chicken, then rub ingredients all over the chicken, be sure to rub inside the cavity as well. Set the chicken on top of the foil balls and set crockpot to high and cook for 8 hrs. Cooking time depends on the size of your chicken. Remove chicken and serve.

Home-style Chicken and Veggie Soup

Servings: 4

2 whole chicken breasts, chopped

4 cup chicken broth

1 whole large onion, chopped

3 whole garlic cloves, minced

8.5 oz. chopped tomatoes

2 whole bell peppers, chopped

1/4 cup cilantro, chopped

1 1/2 cup corn

1 can tomato sauce

1 tsp chili powder

1 tsp cumin powder

1/2 tsp ground black pepper

1 tsp salt

1 lemon

Put the chopped chicken in a crockpot. Add all chopped vegetables and spices to it. Mix well. Cover and cook for 6-8 hrs on low. See the thickness of soup. To adjust the thickness use chicken broth or water. Squeeze some lime juice all over and serve! Enjoy the soup with a byte of veggies or chicken in every sip.

Artichoke & Mushroom Chicken

Servings: 4-6

6 chicken breasts, boneless, halved

8 oz. whole artichoke hearts

8 oz. whole mushrooms, halved

8 oz. marinated artichoke hearts with liquid

1/2 cup balsamic vinegar

1 ½ tsp. Paprika powder

Spread whole artichokes over bottom of Crock-Pot. Add half of mushrooms. Layer chicken over mushrooms. Top chicken with marinated artichoke hearts and their liquid. Add remaining mushrooms. Pour vinaigrette over all ingredients. Cover and cook on low for 4 to 5 hours. Garnish with paprika. Serve in bowl.